The Ultimate Fitness Lifestyle Guide

Brendon Kawondera

Copyright © 2022 by Brendon Kawondera

First printed in 2022 by: Book Printing UK

The right of Brendon Kawondera to be identified as the author of this work has been asserted by him in accordance with the Copyright, Designs and Patents Act 1988.

All Rights Reserved

No reproduction, copy or transmission of this publication may be made without written permission. No paragraph of this publication may be reproduced, copied or transmitted save with the written permission or in accordance with the provisions of the Copyright Act 1956.

ISBN: 978-1-3999-3502-9

Find out more at:

Website: www.btkfitnessandcoaching.com

Email: btkptinfo@gmail.com

Instagram: @btkfitnessandcoaching

CONTENTS

Acknowledgements 4

Why I wrote this book 5

Commitment Statement 6

How to use this book 7

What is the PSP formula? 8

What should I expect? 9

CHAPTER 1: Sleep 11

CHAPTER 2: Stress 19

CHAPTER 3: Work and Education 23

CHAPTER 4: Mood and Attitude (Relationships) 31

CHAPTER 5: Addictions and Cravings (Nutrition) 39

CHAPTER 6: Me Time (Hobbies and Entertainment) 47

CHAPTER 7: Finances (Budgeting and Investing) 53

CHAPTER 8: Planning and Preparation (Daily, Weekly, Monthly, Quarterly, Yearly) 59

CHAPTER 9: Environment and Energy 67

CHAPTER 10: Workout Programs and Structure 73

Acknowledgements

I would like to thank all my clients who contributed to this book with their own unique and special fitness journeys. I thank my mother Abigail, my farther Gilbert, my grandmothers Rebecca Chidziva and Mavis Kawondera, my family, my mentors and my friends. I thank God for blessing me with my son Ezra who is a driving force for all my big dreams.

Why I wrote this book

As a personal trainer I expect everyone to be optimal in all core aspects of their existence in order to positively change their lives and achieve any goals they set themselves. The Priority Checklist of Wellness and Greatness (wealth = health) is an amazing tool which has been very effective with all my clients. From getting the promotion they wanted at work, finding the partner they have been looking for, curing some diseases and living drugs free, stopping smoking, starting their own businesses, to gaining confidence in the gym, losing weight, fat loss, building muscle, becoming financially stable and most importantly becoming happier and healthier.

Helping a handful of people at a time in the gym is great for me, but it's an honour to be able to help many more people in your position on their fitness journey. I am so excited for you to start using this book which has my best methods as a coach. As you embark on your journey you must be proud of yourself because 5% of your purchase is going to help pregnant women, special maternity wards and ambulance services in Zimbabwe. From this day on and for years to come, your life will never be the same again. "I already made the 100% COMMITMENT to help you so now it's your turn!"

Commitment Statement

I ……………………………………….commit to

- Firstly, identify the priorities that I need to work on in order to turn my problems into progressive success.

- Secondly, I will evaluate the solutions and strategies that I implement every 2-4 weeks to monitor my progress.

- Thirdly, I am confident that I will succeed in everything I do because I have eliminated all fear and doubt in myself. I deserve a great life.

For this book to work:

If you do nothing, nothing happens. As soon as you identify the priorities, make your mind up to act immediately. There is NO room for procrastination. This is where the prioritisation works its magic; it gives you perspective on how you intend to change your life positively.

Golden rule – Trust your body, it has the power to heal itself. "Healthy body, healthy mind and a joyful soul."

How to use this book

Now you have made your mind up to live life to the fullest and be great. The rules are simple:

1. You carefully pick the priorities based on the (Personal Strategy Planning) PSP evaluation.
2. You need to accept the priorities as they are. Remember "submission is power".
3. Ask yourself the fundamental questions – Who? What? When? Why? and Where?
4. Shift your paradigm – Change your MINDSET.
5. Get to work – Using your own will and intuition follow the suggested solutions or formulate your own strategy.

Note: The PSP evaluation will only work if you are honest with your answers. If something is genuinely a priority, then make it certain you make it one.

A – means its high priority, take immediate action.

B – means medium priority, act after the A list is taken care of.

C – means low priority, address issue after A and B.

What is the PSP formula?
PSP can stand for any of the following

PERSONAL SELF-CARE PACKAGE

PERSONAL STRATEGY PLANNING

PROBLEM SOLVING PERSON

PROBLEMS SOLUTIONS PREPARATION

POWER STRENGTH PERSISTENCE

What should I expect?

After using all the suggested habits, tools and resources you will have a healthy and wealthy lifestyle. From the moment you purchase this book to the day you die you are now equipped with your own tricks, hacks, strategies, strengths and solutions that work for you. This book brings self-discovery, knowledge of self and self-mastery together to give that healthy, wealthy lifestyle that we all crave for.

A healthy relationship with exercise.

You must be aware of body dysmorphia. Body dysmorphic disorder is when you constantly worry about your appearance, so you end setting unrealistic goals based on insecurities and low self-esteem. Don't fall into this dangerous pit of desiring the body that you have seen on the internet which encourages extreme weight loss or extreme muscle gain/bulking caused by chemicals. This is not ideal for the human body. You must respect your body enough to be patient and to wait for the results. You cannot skip the 4-letter word: WORK. Find a balance in everything and stay away from quick-fix chemicals. It is not worth it.

Whenever I mention wealth, I don't mean Elon Musk or Oprah Winfrey or Jay-Z or Warren Buffett's level of money in the bank. But you must agree that all these individuals have a level of genius, and they operate at a frequency of abundance, joy of existence, gratitude, peace and love, all these elevated emotions which make them great.

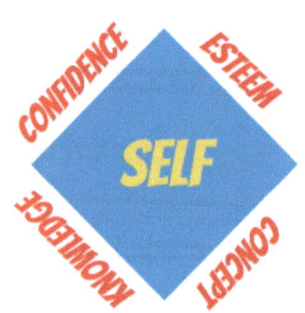

It took me a while to understand when people say, "love yourself". Not everything is going to be perfect, but I believe everyone should be able to experience and appreciate the human body (the vehicle of life) and all its organs functioning all together in perfect harmony. No matter where you are on the Planet Earth, no matter what kind of situation you are in, you are great in your own unique way, and you must celebrate your life every day you wake up.

CHAPTER 1:

Sleep

We all know how **sleep** is so important to us. In today's world, research shows that a lot of people are sleep deprived. I came up with the 5-star bedtime routine when I realised 1 out of 3 of my clients were not getting enough sleep. Sleeping 5/6 hours or less throws off your recovery and hormone balance. More importantly inadequate sleep increases fatigue which affects your performance in the gym or your ability to do daily tasks efficiently. I used to struggle to fall asleep at times but when I focused and concentrated on making sure the process was more efficient, I started sleeping better.

I consider the following as the 3 forms of sleep deprivation:

1. Struggle to fall asleep
2. Struggle to stay asleep
3. Sleep walking / disturbed sleep patterns

The goal should be to have good quality sleep as the research shows that people who a have deep sleep are calmer and happier than people who have poor quality and disturbed sleep. They are more irritable, easily get agitated and they are more stressed. The first step is to be in a good mood, which creates good relationships with people you interact with daily, is by having enough REM (Rapid Eye Movement) sleep.

When it comes to training you must ensure that you maximise your recovery with many techniques out there; like massage, cold therapy etc. During your rest days is when you get stronger. When people ask me for recovery tips I always say, "The best recovery from training is sleep." And obviously nutrition and hydration should be taken care of.

The prioritisation is based on the quality of sleep and the number of hours you get to sleep.

PSP evaluation:

A: 3-5 hours, does not dream, diagnosed insomnia or sleep apnoea.

B: 6-7 hours, cannot remember dreams, wakes up tired, need coffee or shower to get going.

C: 8-9 hours, feels energetic, remembers dreams, fresh mind.

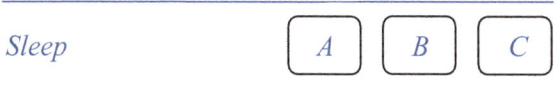

More than 9 hours could be hypersomnia – a condition where you oversleep and feel very tired/sleepy during the day. Visit your doctor or a specialist if this occurs. The only exception for sleeping more than 9 hours to recover are world class athletes who sometimes train at very high intensity and more frequently compared to someone who goes to the gym recreationally once or twice a week. For athletes, sleep is important in order to fully recover.

Solutions:

Track and monitor sleep

Some people prefer not to wear a watch to sleep and that's fine. My mum and many people I know have smart watches, but they do not use them so before you go and purchase one, make it a vow that you will take your time to understand how it works and use it. If you own a watch or can afford to have a smart watch, then you can try using it to track your own sleep and recovery. **Remember, what gets measured gets accomplished.**

Another big issue is the food and drink you consume during the day or before bed that makes you struggle to sleep. Too many caffeinated drinks will keep you wired up and very alert which can make it difficult to relax and rest. If you like a coffee during the day or pre-workout, make sure you drink plenty of water too.

5 STAR BEDTIME ROUTINE

How long does it take?

It takes about 30-45 minutes.

How long shall I do it for?

The 5-star bedtime routine must be followed every night for 30 days.

When shall I do it?

You should set a bedtime reminder on your phone.

5-STAR BEDTIME ROUTINE

30-45 minutes

1. Put a glass of water next to your bed.
2. Write down 10 things you're grateful for.
3. Send love to 3 people bothering you.
4. Ask God or Universe for guidance.
5. Write down 3 important tasks to complete the next day.
6. Read 1 chapter of a self-development book.
7. No light in the room.
8. Turn off all electronics.
9. Mobilise and stretch shoulders and neck.
10. Lay on back, begin deep diaphragmatic breathing.

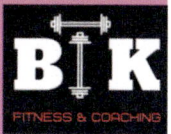

CHAPTER 2:

Stress

Stress kills the body, it destroys the important cells in your body that help you fight infections, viruses and bacteria. Stress management is the biggest and most important factor which needs your full attention. Helping others around you manage their stress will also help you tremendously to reduce and deal with your own stress.

New research shows 34% of people consider their jobs as stressful, health is at 17% and financial problems 30% cause of stress. This is not mentioning environmental stressors which are addressed in Chapter 9 of this book. In this time of uncertainty, the Covid Pandemic, inflation and recession - you must learn to adapt. Take your time when you get to Chapter 7 it has important information on investing, which can help manage stress connected to finances.

I don't like to dwell on stress because as I mention the word 'stress' your brain instantly channels more energy on the actual personal stress that you are individually experiencing. Stress can hinder your *Greatness* lifestyle. So, we will spend little time on this subject before we become vulnerable to thinking that we are stressed and stay on this negative frequency.

You become what you think about, so choose the positive mental attitude.

Key questions

1. Do you consider yourself as a stressed person or have you ever been depressed?

2. What do you do when you're stressed? Do you cook, clean, cry or eat when you're stressed?

Anxiety and worry are separate issues, but they directly affect the overall stress levels.

PSP evaluation:

A: Feel agitated, binge eating, smoke, drink, reactive behaviour.

B: Complain, lets things slide in the moment but moans and rants to colleagues or close ones.

C: Easy going, laid back, responsive behaviour.

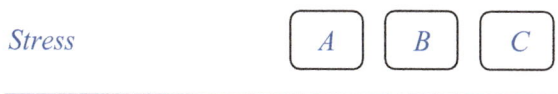

Solutions:

Remember PSP can mean that you are a problem-solving-person. Talk to someone close to you (a personal trainer if you have one or other experts), practise the box breathing technique (4 seconds inhale, 4 seconds exhale), say your positive affirmations, practise manifestation, write a gratitude list, send love to 3 people bothering you, ask God/the Universe for guidance.

If stress is a high priority, if you experience extreme cases of high stressful situations or panic attacks, practise the self-application Cortices Technique by *BodyTalk Founder John Veltheim.*

https://www.youtube.com/watch?v=LqzsfszL4lc&t=22s

Get rid of negative influences. This could be the people you surround yourself with. If they are not helping you, they are bringing you down and you must be aware of them. If you constantly update yourself with world news you are bound to get stressed. Keep news consumption regulated and finely handpicked only for updates and informative debates, even then you must be careful that you don't get engrossed in some of these debates which do not affect your reality. Be present, be aware, breathe and enjoy your great life.

CHAPTER 3:

Work and Education

Throughout our lives we're in education from nursery, pre-school, primary education, secondary or high school, to college, university, masters, PHD, CPD; the list goes on and on. This is a system that we all follow, sometimes not by choice especially before we become teenagers. I'm not knocking down education because it's a vital part of how this world works and we all need to be educated to some degree to be up to date and integrate into society. However, taking a test to see how much you can remember is not a fair representation for any individual's capabilities.

When I was at university studying Sport and Exercise Science, I reached burnout. So, I decided to quit at the end of the second year. My mother and grandmother were not happy with my decision. I spent many hours on the phone with them trying to convince me to go back. My farther on the other hand was supportive of every decision I made, and he was willing to help every single step of the way. The main reasons for my burnout were a lack of concentration on my studies and not getting enough rest from sprinting. Deep down I was also feeling very discouraged for not getting the top grades I wanted.

All I wanted was to be out on the track to train and compete, this is where I felt so alive. Just like at the gym with many other forms of exercise we release endorphins, dopamine and serotonin – the feel-good hormones. All my worries, stress and problems disappeared on the track. My only way out was to self-fund my career in sprinting with the 2020 Tokyo Olympic games in mind, so I thought starting a business would be the best thing I could ever do. I bought my van and self-taught myself how to clean ovens. All I thought of was getting the money. So, I worked out that everyone has an oven in their house, and they probably never have time to clean it properly.

Sunshine Oven-Shine was born in 2017. I cleaned a few ovens with the help of a friend, but within 3 weeks I decided to close the business. I had no fun, no passion and no drive to carry on. Clearly the money wasn't enough. I decided to start a taxi business. I had to learn the maps and memorise key locations and roads of Welwyn and Hatfield boroughs. It took me 30 days to go and take the most difficult test I have had to take in my life. To my surprise I passed. But this proved to me that if you put your mind to something and you have the burning desire you can achieve anything.

Working as a taxi guy opened my eyes to another world. I drove businessmen to the airport, I drove pregnant women to hospitals, I drove children to school, I drove drunk people home in the early hours of the morning, I drove recovered patients from the hospital. I had very interesting conversations with everyone I met. The most interesting thing that always happened was that before most people got out of my taxi, they would ask how old I was.

Every time I answered, "I am 24 years old," they would all tell me to go back to school to study something. I didn't always admit that I had quit university and for months to come I would ponder on this matter thinking what would happen if I went back to study. The main lesson I took from this job was that everyone has the choice to live the life they want to live. After 6 months I quit the taxi business and went back to university and finished my degree.

I made my mother very proud. On my return to university, I had a positive mindset and attitude which meant that I was calmer and my approach towards education was a better one. Looking back now my 2020 Tokyo Olympic dream/vision would have been disrupted by the Covid pandemic and I would have had to adapt and survive. You never know what life may throw at you. Stopping sprinting was difficult but this was just one door closing and a bigger one opened, but the key is that I am still doing what I love.

In total I had 16 jobs. I got promoted in most of them, but I could not see myself working for someone else and taking orders all day and being easily replaced if one day I fell ill. Some people do not mind working under someone's supervision and not taking on 100% responsibility – that is ok. But I decided to take the entrepreneurial route. Never start working purely in the pursuit of money. If you commit to a job, make sure you do it well to reach your goal and create the life you want to live. I pursued a career in athletics and football. I learnt many lessons from it. I am still on this journey just like everybody else.

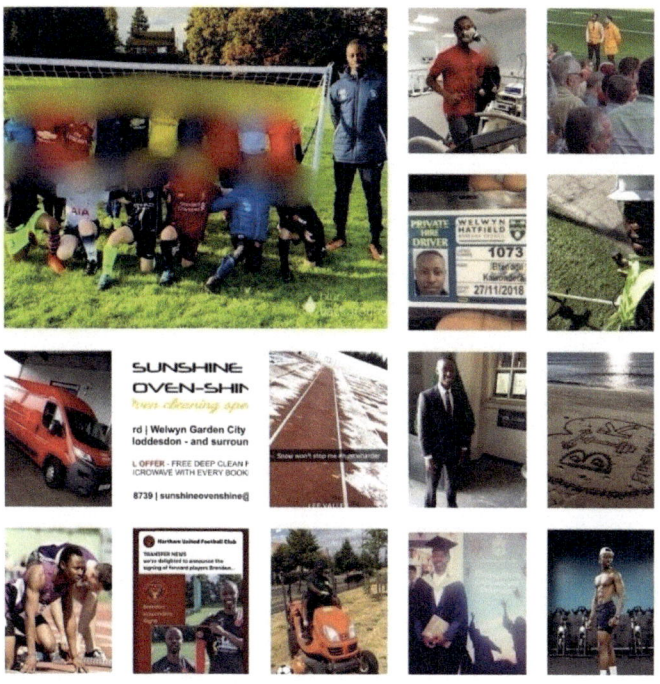

PSP evaluation:

Work related

A: Burnout (usually overworks, doesn't get enough credit, people pleasing, struggling to fit in with colleagues and ready to quit).

B: Just surviving (wants to change jobs, wants promotion, has an exit plan).

C: Personal enjoyment and satisfaction (very happy with work, energised at work).

Education related

A: Burnout (never has enough time to study, exams get overwhelming, fear of failure, ego gets in the way to ask for help).

B: Finds studying stressful but wants to push and put in a good effort to achieve desired grade.

C: Personal enjoyment: on target with grades and assignments, interested in the subject.

| Work & Education | A | B | C |

Solutions:

The goal is to match your desires to the way you live your life. What directly affects me now is that things are always changing in the fitness industry. If you're not careful you will be left behind. You will find yourself trying to coach people that know more than you do and that's not a good position to be in, so I continuously seek out new knowledge and research in the industry.

If you are in a job, I suggest that you work hard every single day. Apply yourself - give 100%. There is power that comes from the four-letter word WORK.

I would hate for anyone to go round in circles like I did, not knowing what they want to do. I obviously look at my job journey as a blessing because I tried many different industries and I now have transferable skills for life. But I recently got introduced to a specific test which reveals your strengths. This will make it so much easier to pick the right job which uses your strengths as an individual so you can live to your unique full potential.

https://www.gallup.com/cliftonstrengths

Use your HR team if you are in burnout at work.

If you are studying and you sense burnout or feel lost, utilise the student support team. If you are not sure about what you really want, take time out. Travel, move away from your local city, discover new things and take your time to really think about what is important to you.

SEEK KNOWLEDGE AND APPLY IT!!!

CHAPTER 4:

Mood and Attitude
(Relationships)

Our mood is majorly affected positively or negatively by the relationships we have with people we interact with. It could be anyone: your partner, boss at work, neighbours, parents, children or friends. This is because we care about how we are perceived within society. Being part of a community is very important for every human being. Fitness classes or team sports clubs are a great way to increase exercise adherence and get involved in social activities regardless of your skill level.

Humans have on average 75 thousand thoughts a day and most of them are what we were thinking about the day before. In order to be great and be in a good mood you must be aware of the thoughts that you have. Take control, don't let your mind control you – you control those thoughts. I like how *Dr Joe Dispenza puts it: "The same thoughts lead to the same choices. The same choices lead to the same behaviour and the same behaviour creates the same experience. The same experience produces the same emotion."*

In order to be in a good mood and have great workouts in the gym or have a good day at work or college, you must be in a positive and vibrant mood. It is difficult to be in a good mood when things are going wrong in your life but if you love yourself and you are grateful for your existence this process becomes easier.

In the past I was fortunate enough to work with a couple who had issues which needed to be worked on. Just working on their mood alone raised self-awareness to control their thoughts and feelings. The self-perception of their thoughts and feelings ultimately led to less arguments and a more joyous relationship. Not to say they now have a near perfect relationship, but sometimes if we are in a bad mood we just want to be heard. **Good communication is vital.**

Another one of my clients was a lady who wanted a promotion at work. She had worked for this company for a very long time. She had gained respect amongst colleagues; however, a few times other colleagues would get the role she wanted. To make matters worse she got complacent when someone else from another company applied for the same job and they got it!

Left in despair, she became resentful, and she almost gave up. I knew how much this job meant to her. So, I encouraged her to work on a positive mood and attitude towards her management team. Obviously, the correct program which consisted of numerous boxing rounds did the trick some days, but a bespoke training program with the right exercises, recovery and nutrition was taken care of first. Suddenly, she started building those broken-down relationships with the people at work, turning up to work with a different mindset. Like a light switch her mood switched from this sad, lethargic, unenthusiastic individual to a joyful, cheerful, positive individual. This energy was very powerful around the office when she walked in. Within 3 months she got promoted to her desired position.

I train a lot of female clients and a big factor which affects their mood is the menstrual cycle. I am not a woman, so my articulation might be limited but this advice I'm about to give on this subject is based on how my clients are. The period affects all women differently. Certainly, some of my clients can train throughout the cycle, and some will find it very difficult.

My advice is to take it easy during those days and try not to be so harsh on yourself. Instead, let nature take its course. The only thing to avoid is feeling too sorry for yourself and start blaming everything on the hormones. You must have the will to fight for the things you really want and not get side-tracked by the temporary or those mood swings.

PSP evaluation:

A: Holding grudges, not letting go of ex, depressed and anxious.

B: Trying to resolve issues seeking help.

C: Patient, grateful, energetic and happy.

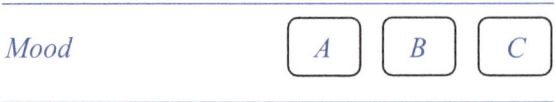

Solutions:

Self-awareness is important. To build emotional intelligence one must deal with emotional issues passionately by setting intentional goals of realising self-worth, self-image and gratitude.

Daily task:

1. Write down 10 things you are grateful for.

2. Send love to 3 people who are bothering you.

3. Ask God/the Universe for guidance.

Music is one of the greatest healers which can lift your mood when you feel stuck. Find some songs that lift you up; make a playlist and keep it on standby like a super sub in a football game.

Having a balanced diet also keeps you in a good mood. The gut brain axis is a strong connection that our food directly affects our brain and how we think. Whenever you find yourself complaining or blaming things or people, stop and think about having something healthy to eat or drink. Other recovery techniques such as cold showers, ice bath, massage, acupuncture, a shiatsu treatment or bath salts are all different methods to lift your mood.

This book is about self-mastery and knowledge of self. I recommend doing a bit of research and find out more about your brain and how it operates. For instance, look up right vs left brain thinking. The right brain which is responsible for emotional expression is more active so you may start feeling jealous, happy, satisfaction or frustration. The left brain is more logical, factual, analytical... This is all free information which can help you elevate and level up in your own unique manner.

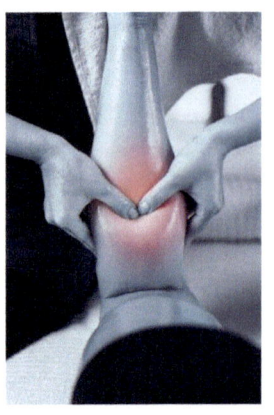

Fellas, if your woman has period cramps you can help her and ladies a quick remedy for period cramps, aches and pain. Your body is its own universe interconnected with many systems, substances and structures. There are some acupressure and reflexology points which can help in many ways to alleviate pain, instantly improve flexibility and in some cases improve strength. For example, there is a point in the centre of your calf muscle. If pressed for about 20 seconds the period pain should stop. Some points along the elbow, foot, ankle, ear and hand can instantly improve strength. Do your research on reflexology and find ways to help yourself without depending on pain killers or chemicals. Some people are more sensitive than others so these techniques might or might not work.

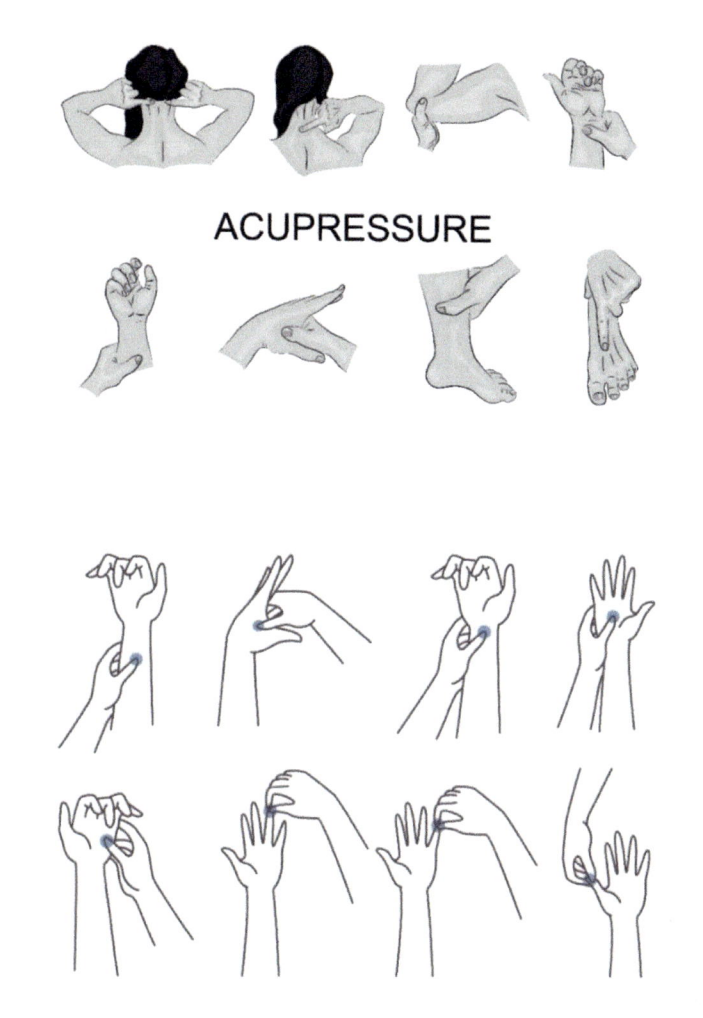

ACUPRESSURE

For more information on instant strength and mobility, get in touch with *Carlos Castro* an incredible mentor of mine.
https://strength-community.com/

CHAPTER 5:

Addictions and Cravings (Nutrition)

Addiction: a chronic dysfunction of the brain system that involves reward, motivation and memory.

Craving: a characteristic of an addictive disorder.

Nobody ever wakes up one day and says I want to get addicted to something. Addiction just happens when one fails to control one's mind and conquer the urges that the body emotionally leads them to. Many addictions can lead to serious health implications, for example the consumption of junk foods can lead to excess body fat or obesity. An addiction to refined sugars will ultimately lead to type 2 diabetes. A caffeine addiction can cause high stress levels, adrenal fatigue or chronic fatigue. Alcohol abuse can lead to kidney disease, cancers and liver cirrhosis.

I believe at some point during lockdown I became addicted to alcohol, but two events turned my life around. Firstly, was when I contracted the Coronavirus; I became so weak to the point I thought I wasn't going to wake up the next day. My immune system was weakened by the alcohol consumption. I knew I was addicted because after my recovery from the virus, I carried on drinking even more.

Other bad things happened in my relationship. When I remembered one incident of a drunk couple who argued in the back of my taxi at the end of a boozy night, I realised how people acted foolishly when drunk. The fondness for such behaviour made me approach a life coach. I am very grateful to have had a life coach who helped me with my problem and changed my life positively. I never acted as this fool again. At first it was difficult to admit that I was dependent on alcohol. I had to genuinely surrender because I wanted more for myself and my family.

What my life coach had done was simple but very effective. She asked a very strong question. She asked me if I wanted my son to grow up and know his father as an alcoholic. My answer to this was a firm NO. For this reason, I decided to change my life for good. Ever since then I am very mindful about my relationship with alcohol.

There are other addictions, the most common are social media, smoking and cravings for sweet things. I remember talking about the mice experiment where some mice were given two paths. The first path led to a very addictive substance (cocaine). The second path led to some sugar. The mice favoured the sugar more. To prove the sugar addiction an electric current was put on the second path which led to the sugar. Still the mice were willing to go through the pain just to get the reward of that sweet tasting sugar.

Everyone can enjoy some sweet food, but a critical self-evaluation on whether your sweet tooth is going to have an adverse effect on your future health is necessary. Excess consumption of sweets and refined sugars causes tooth decay, weight gain, diabetes, some cancers, lowers testosterone, and spikes insulin which can cause mood swings.

PSP evaluation:

A: Must have a sweet dessert, needs to smoke, withdrawal symptoms from stimulants, unusual agitated and anger, finally failure to admit addiction.

B: Can quit easily but relapses all the time, getting help, cutting down, looking for healthy alternatives.

C: Feels normal not taking any stimulants, not reliant and has a balanced diet.

Addiction & Cravings	A	B	C

Solutions:

When I deal with clients who have addictions such as smoking, sex, food, social media, work, shopping or exercise, I introduce them to the wheel of change which encompasses all stages of change. It helps massively if you become aware of what stage you are on. The other big factor is recognising your physical environment. Your environment affects your mental state. There are triggers all around you and it all comes down to how you plan and structure your daily routines which can make you change positively to an addiction free life.

Intentionally ask yourself why you started in the first place!!

Wheel of change:

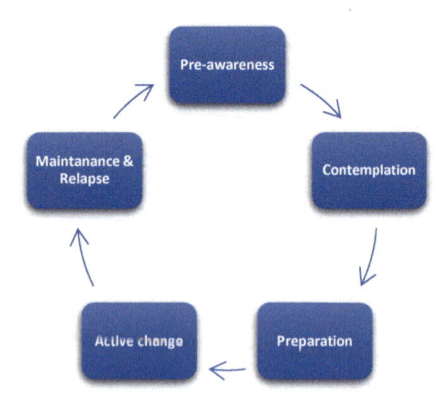

Pre-awareness → Contemplation → Preparation → Active change → Maintanance & Relapse → (back to Pre-awareness)

Nowadays it is easy to get addicted to fast food because the shops are around every corner. If you want good health, you must have a balanced diet

Your relationship with food

1. Try your best to eat organic – the cheapest isn't always the best.
2. Prepare your meals, get familiar with cooking.
3. Eat specific foods for specific times. (Rainbow on your plate – colourful vegitables.)
4. Monitor how you feel after eating certain foods.
5. Drink enough water.

"How you eat tells your genes what type of body you want later." Dharma Singh Khalsa

Many people on their fitness journey want help with their nutrition. I always have people who ask me how I manage to keep my body lean. The answer is simple, MODERATION. To achieve a balanced weight and look a certain way you must have a balanced diet. If you are in bad shape, you must first accept that you need to work hard, and it will be difficult at the beginning, but when you start seeing results the journey becomes easier to maintain as a lifestyle. Some people like to point fingers and blame things on genetics or age or time. All these are excuses which never get you anywhere.

The formula is simple:

If you want to lose weight clean your diet (no to soul foods), eat less and move more.

If you want to build muscle eat healthy, hit your macronutrient goals and lift heavy.

Vitamins and minerals – you must have an adequate number of fruits and vegetables.

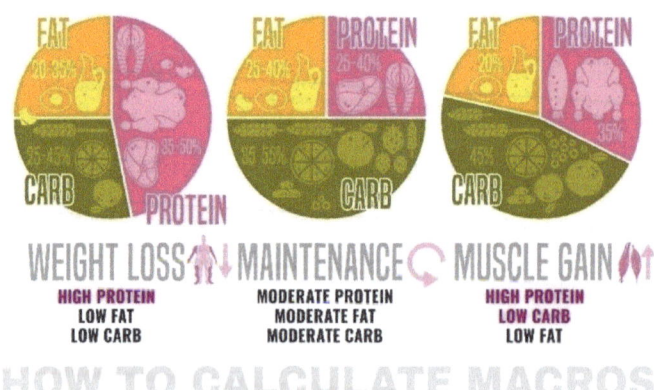

Some people like to count calories, some people don't. Calories are a grey area because it is dependent on age, weight, height, activity levels, occupation and access to food labelling etc.

Online calorie calculator:
https://www.bodybuilding.com/fun/macronutcal.htm

CHAPTER 6:

Me Time

(Hobbies and Entertainment)

Many people ask me why I am always smiling. This is because my gratitude bar is so high because of where I come from and what I have been through. I believe everybody must learn the ability to shut down their thoughts and be fully present in the moment.

Me time is a special time where you can re-invent yourself and you don't have to think as much about your problems and daily tasks. It is in this time you need to only allow positive thoughts, love, gratitude, joy and peace. In many religions isolation/limitations/fasting is usually the answer to this. Being alone will allow you time to find out more about yourself.

In terms of stress management, you must plan things that eliminate boredom. Try to change the way you do things. If you hate anything you do that means you are already aware that you can change it, so do something about it. Do things out of curiosity, creativity and imagination.

"The only thing that is ultimately real about your journey, is the step you are taking at this moment. That's all there ever is." Eckhart Tolle

Going to the gym is also me time. When we exercise there is a transmutation of energies felt in that moment or throughout the day. It is important to be aware of your mind state before going to the gym. Exercising can be a great way to relieve stress, but you cannot train every day to dump your worries and forget your problems or act like they don't exist. PSP: become a problem-solving-person and fix things.

Avoid getting addicted to exercise. Have a healthy fitness journey, one that is sustainable and has no addictions. An addiction to exercise is called exercise dependency. Exercise dependency can occur when you are constantly seeking to feel good from hormones like dopamine and serotonin. This can quickly turn into overtraining; the effects of overtraining will lead to injury and ultimately becomes a weakness. This is a slippery slope because you will then feel discouraged to pursue your initial goal and fail to adhere to your training program.

Many people wonder why they are not getting any stronger, faster or leaner even after training most days of the week. If one of the reasons, they are overtraining is due to exercise dependency this can be very difficult to understand. I advise you to get a personal trainer to guide you and motivate you to do the right thing.

PSP evaluation:

A: Never have me time, no time to relax, always on the go.

B: Only attends social activities, needs other people for entertainment.

C: Spends some quality alone time, has an outdoor and indoor hobby, meditates.

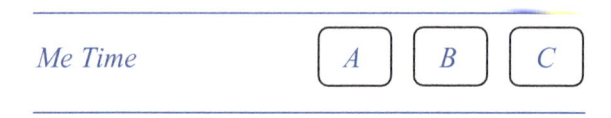

| Me Time | A | B | C |

Solutions:

Taking time out by yourself by going to the park, visiting an art gallery, watching a live band, going to the library, learning a new skill or language etc. These are all things you can schedule into your routine other than just going to the gym or always hanging out with friends.

A good way to figure out what to do during me time is to do things you used to do when you were a child under the age of 13. Why? Because this is when you still had a very imaginative mind, so all play was fun. Even as an adult when you start doing these things you will find childhood memories pop back as nostalgia.

Silence in the middle of chaos. Being alone can be tough for a lot of people but if you think of when you were little baby you were born alone into the world. You would always be doing something because there is so much to learn. I encourage you to study history, art, technology, science, and more importantly studying yourself is a brilliant way to spend me-time. In the beginning doing things by yourself might seem confusing but it will soon get better with time.

In order to enjoy me time you need to install an element of child-like play and fun. It is an important part of our lives which we are connected by, and we can all relate to. When we were babies/toddlers we were always fed and full of energy – we could run up and down throughout the entire day. This is because our nutrition was taken care of, we had enough sleep and good hydration. The only task we had to do was to play. Everything was taken care of by our parents or whoever raised us. In adulthood we might feel a bit lost when those basics are not taken care of due to a lack of responsibility. Therefore, the fundamental part of your fitness journey is to master self-care and connect with those great childhood memories.

"Sometimes just smile and laugh a lot." – Brendon Kawondera

CHAPTER 7:

Finances

(Budgeting and Investing)

Budgeting

About 10 years ago I started using the Barclays mobile banking app. This was completely revolutionary to me because for once I could see the amount of money I had without having to walk or drive to the ATM or wait in a long bank queue to answer a load of security questions to gain access to my account.

Mobile banking brought about a great convenience but also secretly an obsession of constantly checking the app. I would end up making unwise purchases and would spend hours trying to calculate my debts and my income. Sometimes I would spend the money before earning it. Doing daily checks just caused more confusion and unnecessary worry which led to stress. I could compare my banking app to TikTok or Instagram. I lacked financial literacy. But thanks to my cousin who bought me the book 'Rich Dad, Poor Dad' by Robert Kiyosaki, the way I look at money has changed. Nowadays I give thanks to brothers who started EYL *(Earn Your Leisure)* for bringing financial literacy to the masses.

Investing – no risk, no reward

In 2017, I was introduced to Forex trading by a friend, who was making some good profits in the game. I traded some of the money I had saved up working as a shop assistant. I made bit of a profit and lost everything because I was impatient and very emotional at the time. This was my first learning curve. I jumped back in, and we made some profits again during the US presidential elections when Donald Trump became president. We had fun with the whole process so now it was time to get in the big league.

My friend discovered a top trader in the city of London. This guy had a seminar going on where he would recruit traders and make more money with them. The seminar was in a grand hotel in central London on one cold evening. We drove into London, parked the car outside the congestion zone to save some money and walked the rest of the way. As we approached the hotel, I could see all these luxurious sports cars. The lobby welcome was very lavish. I began to feel rich.

During the introduction the main man made sure he pointed out which one of those cars was his. It was the James Bond Casino Royale Aston Martin.

The presentation was perfected to a T, he showed us all the figures and proof so that every single person in the audience was convinced that they could become millionaires and it was going to take them less than a year to do so. My friend went ahead and signed up at the end of the workshop. He made some profits, and he is still making money and losing money in trading.

During the conference I realised my goal was a little bit different to most people in the audience. I realised that money is never yours to keep, it will always come and go. No matter how much you have, you can lose it all and make it all back again. The idea is to not get emotionally attached to it. It was this day that I made a choice to only invest in myself. I am not saying don't trade because you can really make a living from it, but you just need to have a strong reason as to WHY you are doing it. When you answer the WHY you have nothing else to worry about.

The fast cars and the nice clothes did not impress me that much and I did not enjoy sitting on a computer screen, sweating and panicking every day about losing money. Hence I do what I do - which is to help people build good relationships and watch them reach their full potential.

PSP Evaluation:

A: Doesn't know where the money is going, checks bank every other day, no savings and struggling to make payments.

B: Trying to manage savings, researching about investments, taking risks

C: Diversified portfolio, has savings, doesn't worry about money, taking calculated risks

Finances	A	B	C

Solutions:

Budgeting: Set aside 30 minutes on one day of the month where you can do your own accounts and balance the income and outgoings. If it's not balanced, formulate a plan of action to sort out the issues and execute. The best tip on budgeting is to pay yourself first at least 20% of your income, spend 20% on living expenses, give 10% to a charity and invest 50%.

Investing: Your mind is the best real estate on earth so I would suggest you invest in yourself. Enrol onto a course or buy some self-help books. My favourite book is 'Think and Grow Rich' by Napoleon Hill, I have read it 3 times now and the book is not about money.

"Time is more valuable than money, you can get more money, but you cannot get more time." Jim Rohn

CHAPTER 8:

Planning and Preparation (Daily, Weekly, Monthly, Quarterly, Yearly)

Planning is a fundamental step in all worthwhile activities, but without dismissing the beauty of spontaneity which brings its own level of discovery and tranquillity, knowing that sometimes things will go the way they do without any human influence. "It is what it is." Some people are good at planning, and they will work better with a pre-existing plan put in place. My plan was to go to the 2020 Olympics. This never happened, but I managed to move on from it.

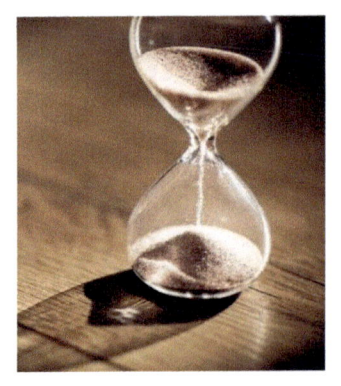

A lot of people on their fitness journey make excuses about not training or failing to prepare their meals. The number one excuse that I hear is a lack of TIME. Nobody really manages time, because time stops for nobody, but you are in full control of the activities you choose to do with your 24 hours. It's up to you as an individual to prioritise significant activities which take you to your goal.

Here is a picture of my whiteboard layout.

Goals	Daily Targets	Gratitude
• 3 months • 6 months • 12 months	1. Meeting with mentor 2. Follow ups 3. Laundry	1. Speaking new language 2. Client reached goal 3. Son growing healthy
Mantra for the week	there is a season for everything	

Notes:

Big reason **WHY**
Helping people realise their full potential in the gym and in their day to day life.
Healing the body from the top down not the bottom up.

Goals	Daily Targets	Gratitude
• • •	1. 2. 3.	1. 2. 3.
Mantra for the week		

Notes:

Big reason **WHY** !

When I discuss personal goals with a client for the very first time, for example weight loss, by the end of the consultation the client leaves my desk with 3 or 5 additional goals that we set according to what takes priority. The prioritisation is what makes the difference between a client that gets results and a client who may feel stuck and feels like they are not making any progress. It is very important that you pinpoint the ONE thing that needs your attention and deal with it promptly. PSP formula – Problem Strategy Preparation – is the key here because when we heal the body, we heal from the head down to the toes, not the bottom up.

"Whatever the mind of men can conceive and believe, the man can achieve with a positive mental attitude." Napoleon Hill

PSP evaluation:

A: No time to cook, misses important deadlines, no diary, always late and procrastinates.

B: On time sometimes, makes excuses, trying to plan and organise.

C: Uses an app for planning, uses a physical diary, meets deadlines and plans meals ahead.

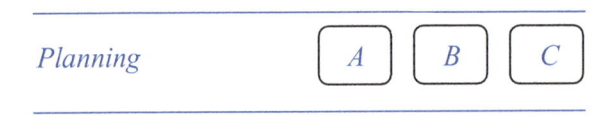

Planning	A	B	C

Solutions:

Daily – We all plan for work, school, holiday or meetings. On your fitness journey there should be a higher level of detail that goes into planning your meals on a day-to-day basis. The key is that food is a necessity for survival and your body will always need the fuel in order to carry on going efficiently - full of energy. Not saying you need to be counting calories and get obsessive over the numbers, but a visit back to Chapter 5 will help.

Weekly – The classic gym attendance trend is that on Mondays the gyms are fully packed. The drop-off rate increases as the week commences. This doesn't come as a surprise because when I look at most people's workout programs there is a lack of appropriate goal setting, and most programs are boring which makes it difficult to stay consistent. For example, the guys like to hit chest and arms and for girls it's glutes and butt. To encourage consistency and adherence I always advise them to:

1. Follow a programme which addresses personal weaknesses with various exercises.
2. Make sure the Friday workout includes their favourite exercises.
3. Start the week off with the boring but fundamental exercises.
4. Train their favourite muscle group on the day they are more likely to skip a gym session.
5. Get a personal trainer to create accountability.

Monthly – Setting yourself 30-day goals is a great way to keep track and monitor progress. Your body is constantly changing and ageing so keep in mind that your level of fitness is always fluctuating. There are many standardised tests for endurance, flexibility, speed, agility and strength that you can easily do in the gym to compare your data with the norms. The set of 30-day goals is to also have other measurements for body composition to check muscle mass, body fat percentage, body weight and muscle imbalances. If you want to take things up a notch you can have blood works test and check for a balance in vitamins, minerals and hormones.

Quarterly – Everyone must make it a goal to travel. By travel I don't mean go out of budget and fly abroad on a lush holiday. It could be visiting a city in your country that you have never been to. We all get the same 12 months in a year. Plan to visit a new place at least once every 4 months. I once heard someone say travelling is like a DNA upgrade. Travelling will lift your spirits but you must go away with an open mind ready to explore. By having these 4 trips you will always have something to look forward to.

Yearly – You are the captain of the ship so taking charge and setting sail is a journey filled with hope. For every year you must have a goal and a plan written down. We all have new year resolutions but not many people get to complete or stick to their new exciting goals. The best and simple way if you do not already know it is to set SMART goals. Specific, Measurable, Attainable, Relevant and Timebound.

Whatever goal you set yourself, be ambitious but grateful at the same time.

CHAPTER 9:

Environment and Energy

Your environment directly affects your energy. You have the power to change and control your environment in order to tap into your greatness and live a fulfilled life. Study your environment and the people you surround yourself with; see if your goals and desires match them.

Bedroom/place of rest:

The first chapter (Sleep) I put emphasis on sleep. It is very important to have a room where there is little to no light when you fall asleep. Your eyes are like the door or window to the world. Your eyes and your brain simultaneously work together to initiate the release of a hormone called melatonin when you are exposed to darkness. Melatonin helps your body clock which helps you fall asleep. The opposite happens when you rise in the morning to the sunlight – your body releases more serotonin.

The position of your pillow, your mattress age, the covers you have over you, the pyjamas you wear (if you wear any), open or closed window, air conditioning or fan and other electronic gadgets, these are all things which must be carefully looked at and assessed to ensure you have a good night's sleep.

Car or public transport: If you drive your car to and from work or commute with the metro/bus/train you must be aware of how you feel. Usually, most people doing the early commute are sleep deprived. So many drivers make mistakes and on public transport people may bump and push into you. Don't take it personally, you are just one human being amongst a billion just navigating through this journey of life. If you remember Chapter 1, not having enough hours of sleep can sometimes cause distress. Sometimes you might find people coming across as rude, unapologetic or ignorant. This is when becoming a great person really counts because you cannot control everything that happens around you, but you can control how you feel or react about any situation.

News and social media: I used to read the news every single day on my phone as soon as I woke up. With today's technology it's super easy for news to spread when something happens somewhere in the world. Due to the Earth having different time zones, the news becomes 24 hours. I would say for myself my brain only focused on the negative news, thought that's not to say there is any good news. When we become empathetic but helpless about a headline, we see on the news our subconscious feels the pain even if we are not actually experiencing the pain ourselves. For example, hearing about mass murders instils fear which leads to a lot of negative emotions. Negative or low vibration frequencies ultimately lead to stress and disease.

Dealing and having conversations with more than 200 gym members every week you can imagine the amount of people

I talk to daily. That number does not include my own personal clients who I must connect with on a deeper level. A lot of people speak negatively most of the time; sometimes without even realising. It's not their fault, sometimes it's just their frequency, so when I talk to people I always filter, control and lead the conversations to my frequency and vibration of positivity.

With any given conversation there is a listener and a speaker at any given moment. With the news or social media, you are just a listener or observer, so you must be aware of the onslaught of information by the algorithm to your subconscious mind, which is unable to filter anything unlike the conscious mind. So, it is very crucial that you become a high-level observer.

"A high-level observer controls what they see, but a low-level observer is controlled by what they see." 19 Keys

PSP evaluation:

A: New apps, peak hour travel, friends who don't inspire you, bad morning routine and reactive.

B: Hears news from other people, cannot control what's coming in.

C: Aware of incoming information, emotionally intelligent.

Environnent & Energy | A | B | C |

Solutions:

Find a good gym, get a personal trainer, join a club or class. Sometimes I consider gym and recreational leisure centres as mental health institutions. Social media and news will never go away and not all news is bad news but be aware of some updates which directly impact you, your family or community. Other people also just like to ponder upon debates, but just remember to be a high-level observer.

Music and laughter can nourish the mind and soul. Listen to some tunes and discover new genres to distract yourself from bad energy. If you followed the Chapter 6 strategies, you should already be better at managing your energy. Your body will not heal itself or live up to its full potential if there is a chakra is blockage. Chakra refers to a spiritual energy centre. The 7 centres are: root, sacral, solar plexus, heart, throat, third eye and crown. Some of the causes of blockages are bad news consumption, trauma, ungratefulness, reactive behaviour or bad energy people. These are all modifiable factors you can work on in order to be great. Chakra clearing meditation are good, lots of guided ones out there online.

CHAPTER 10:

Workout Programs and Structure

Disclaimer: All forms of exercise can help with all kinds of physiological, psychological and physical states you are in. The execution of any given workout may vary based on the desired goal and the individual's ability. Ability extension comes from several experiments I have tried and tested on myself and my clients over time and got results.

This is one of my favourite chapters because this is where you get to learn the fundamentals of creating your own training program and how to structure it according to your needs. I did not provide a workout program in this book to give you flat stomach or 6-pack abs or a peachy bum or to get rid of the bingo wings. This is because there is more that goes into designing a bespoke training program that produces results.

Anyone that I work with first completes several tests including the main Braverman test. If you are interested in working with me, sign up on my website

www.btkfitnessandcoaching.com

Here are some **FAQs** which may help you on your fitness journey:

Is there any pill or supplement to get my dream body?

EXERCISE is the number 1 pill/drug out there on the market and the sooner you understand how your body works the quicker you will become confident. The more confident you are in yourself the better your fitness journey will be and the better you will perform in any sport you participate in or in general fitness in the gym.

How do I design a training program?

Needs analysis is the first step to designing a good fitness program that will address the issues at hand and allow you to reach your goal. Set your fitness goals in the same way I described setting SMART goals in Chapter 8. For more help with some of the best program design, I recommend getting in touch with Julian Ernst

https://www.tempoperformance.com/

Is there limit to what I can do in the gym?

A fit body is one that has good, not extreme flexibility, strength, agility, speed, coordination, balance and endurance, except in some cases of disabilities caused by accidents, injuries or deformities from birth.

"No Limit" Ash Atour.

How long shall I train for?

Many people struggle to find enough time to train, so to get over this hurdle I suggest that you check out my video on how to plan effectively and execute in just 60 minutes.

https://www.youtube.com/watch?v=FvmmS_d6z_0

For females: Shall I train on my period?

Nobody works like a robot; our energy levels and emotions are constantly fluctuating. It is mandatory to always check in with my clients about how they are feeling. As for females I always keep in mind that they could be on their period. The awareness of such times allows me to adapt and customise the session for them.

For women in menopause or experiencing PMS – your hormones may be all over the place. You might feel a bit confused and not know what to do sometimes. My advice is always to listen to your body. Every woman is different. Some of my clients can train throughout their period although their strength levels may be lower than usual, they still get on with training. Some female clients might feel very weak, and they just want to rest and recover; this is also ok. It is important to understand that you must be patient on your fitness journey. It is endless and you must always train in anticipation of things like injury, illness and other circumstances.

Another interesting part is the magical moment of conceiving and remaining fit during pregnancy. I am not an expert in training pregnant woman. I always refer mothers-to-be to my fellow trainers who specialise in this area. If you are expecting I suggest you get as much help as you can from experts and use the resources out there to maintain your fitness and give your baby/babies a good chance of a healthy gestation period.

For males:

Does stress affect performance or erectile dysfunction?

We are gifted that our bodies naturally produce more testosterone. Testosterone helps to maintain muscle mass and strength. Stress is one of the main testosterone killers, along with certain medications, refined sugars, inactivity and excess body fat. Men, simply be mellow and manage your stress and you should be ok.

Can I boost testosterone production?

Aim for semen retention for 2-4 weeks or even longer depending on your circumstances. If you abstain from sex or ejaculating, you will see an increase in strength. Everyone's threshold is different, but remember this book is about you becoming a master of self. Doing certain exercises also boosts testosterone and growth hormones; I recommend heavy sled push and pull, leg press, squat, bench and deadlift.

I struggle to fall asleep, what time shall I train?

I strongly suggest that you train in the morning instead of the night. Why? Raising your heart rate before bedtime could be a bad thing if you do not produce enough melatonin or

GABA (Gamma-aminobutyric acid). This is because GABA is an inhibitory neurotransmitter which blocks or reduces the activity of the central nervous system (CNS).

For example, if you are in a heightened state like dancing to loud music or boxing where you release a lot of adrenaline or lifting very heavy weights, your CNS is overactive. It will take you awhile to calm down and decrease the resting heart rate and bring it down closer to the sleeping range. Compare this to someone who is calm because they just finished doing yoga or having a massage; they are more likely to fall asleep quicker.

Shall I train by myself?

This depends partially on the type of person you are, introvert or extrovert. If you are new to training, I believe having a training partner, joining a class or hiring personal trainer is a great way to lift your mood and have a better exercise experience.

Ability Extension

The best tools to maximise your training sessions are visualisation, self-talk, music and willpower. If you put these together with a calm mind you may experience a "FLOW" state or "being in the zone". I experienced this whenever I ran my fastest race or scored some goals on the football pitch and just celebrated but didn't know how much of it was a fluke.

When you turn up for a session at the gym or park or even at home:

- "Stand with your back straight, chest out and shoulders back."
- "Inhale for 2 seconds through your nose and exhale through your mouth for 2 seconds."
- "Begin to visualise the strongest version of yourself."
- "Visualise the most confident version of yourself."
- "Visualise the happiest version of yourself."
- "Make every single rep count."

In this moment you must become that person you want to be. The self-talk from then on is what will change you. You must declare that you are strong and that you can execute the moves correctly. Nowadays people use the term BEAST but I love the bible verse that says, "I can do all things through Christ who strengthens me." Philippians 4: 11-13

During a workout your brain is very active, and it sends so many neurons (information messengers) across the entire body. This mechanism is there to help you enhance your motor skills. You can maximise it by the type of music you choose to listen to in that moment. I want you to perform like the biggest star of the show. Enter the "flow" state, which is the highest form of confidence and where doing something seems effortless. The more you frequently enter this state where afterwards you feel a great sense of joy, reward and rush of dopamine, the more positive you will become.

The flow state is a key to a life full of GREATNESS.

When I'm coaching, I shout words of encouragement because I know sometimes, we all need to turn on that switch and crank things up to kickstart the inner belief. Trusting your body when doing those challenging exercises is the beginning of ability extension. Never underestimate willpower, it is one of the supernatural powers that God gave us. Willpower plus the tactical self-talk can unlock your hidden potential.

I hope this book positively changes your life and the lives of your loved ones too. Keep an eye out for volume 2.

Week 1

CHECKLIST TO GREATNESS AND WELLNESS

	A	B	C
SLEEP - (5* bedtime routine)	☐	☐	☐
STRESS - (clean, cook, cry, eat)	☐	☐	☐
WORK / EDUCATION - (personal enjoyment and burnout)	☐	☐	☐
MOOD - (relationships)	☐	☐	☐
ADDICTIONS / CRAVINGS - (nutrition)	☐	☐	☐
ME TIME - (hobbies and entertainment)	☐	☐	☐
FINANCES - (budgeting and investing)	☐	☐	☐
PLANNING - (daily, weekly, monthly, quarterly, yearly)	☐	☐	☐
ENVIRONMENT - (bedroom, noise, car, music, newspaper, news, friends)	☐	☐	☐

A GOAL WITHOUT A PLAN IS JUST A WISH.....

A - High priority, major significance
B - Medium priority, medium significance
C - Low priority, minor significance

Week 4

CHECKLIST TO GREATNESS AND WELLNESS

	A	B	C
SLEEP - (5* bedtime routine)	☐	☐	☐
STRESS - (clean, cook, cry, eat)	☐	☐	☐
WORK / EDUCATION - (personal enjoyment and burnout)	☐	☐	☐
MOOD - (relationships)	☐	☐	☐
ADDICTIONS / CRAVINGS - (nutrition)	☐	☐	☐
ME TIME - (hobbies and entertainment)	☐	☐	☐
FINANCES - (budgeting and investing)	☐	☐	☐
PLANNING - (daily, weekly, monthly, quarterly, yearly)	☐	☐	☐
ENVIRONMENT - (bedroom, noise, car, music, newspaper, news, friends)	☐	☐	☐

A GOAL WITHOUT A PLAN IS JUST A WISH.....

A - High priority, major significance
B - Medium priority, medium significance
C - Low priority, minor significance

Week 8

CHECKLIST TO GREATNESS AND WELLNESS

	A	B	C
SLEEP - (5* bedtime routine)	☐	☐	☐
STRESS - (clean, cook, cry, eat)	☐	☐	☐
WORK / EDUCATION - (personal enjoyment and burnout)	☐	☐	☐
MOOD - (relationships)	☐	☐	☐
ADDICTIONS / CRAVINGS - (nutrition)	☐	☐	☐
ME TIME - (hobbies and entertainment)	☐	☐	☐
FINANCES - (budgeting and investing)	☐	☐	☐
PLANNING - (daily, weekly, monthly, quarterly, yearly)	☐	☐	☐
ENVIRONMENT - (bedroom, noise, car, music, newspaper, news, friends)	☐	☐	☐

A GOAL WITHOUT A PLAN IS JUST A WISH.....

A - High priority, major significance
B - Medium priority, medium significance
C - Low priority, minor significance

Week 12

CHECKLIST TO GREATNESS AND WELLNESS

	A	B	C
SLEEP - (5* bedtime routine)	☐	☐	☐
STRESS - (clean, cook, cry, eat)	☐	☐	☐
WORK / EDUCATION - (personal enjoyment and burnout)	☐	☐	☐
MOOD - (relationships)	☐	☐	☐
ADDICTIONS / CRAVINGS - (nutrition)	☐	☐	☐
ME TIME - (hobbies and entertainment)	☐	☐	☐
FINANCES - (budgeting and investing)	☐	☐	☐
PLANNING - (daily, weekly, monthly, quarterly, yearly)	☐	☐	☐
ENVIRONMENT - (bedroom, noise, car, music, newspaper, news, friends)	☐	☐	☐

A GOAL WITHOUT A PLAN IS JUST A WISH....

A - High priority, major significance
B - Medium priority, medium significance
C - Low priority, minor significance

Progress

	Week 1	Week 4	Week 8	Week 12
Weight loss				
Muscle gain				
Maintenance				
Body fat %				

Notes:

Notes: